Made for This

Birthing Essentials from a Former Labor and Delivery Nurse and Mother of Two

Contents:

Introduction

I was 22 years old and had just landed my dream job. I was honored to have accepted a Labor and Delivery Registered Nurse position at the reputable University of Kansas Hospital. I'll never forget my first shift when every bed was full, and we had no choice but to line the hallways with laboring moms in wheelchairs. We had interpreters standing by to help assess and care for several of these families that were not fluent in English. I bravely began triaging with clipboard in hand and somehow made it through that first night. When I started there, all births were done in the operating rooms. Women would labor, and even begin pushing, in their private room until the doctor determined she was within minutes of delivery. Then, it was a mad dash to the operating room, often with a sheet loosely flung over the laboring mom and a nurse sitting on the end of the bed. Those first few births were both intense and absolutely magical. I often wondered if I would ever witness a birth without tears welling in my eyes.

As a new nurse, I soaked in the "method" of how labor was done in a university hospital environment without realizing there was any other way or perspective on how to labor and birth. I had learned "the drill." I knew how to quickly and efficiently assess the woman in the bed while simultaneously placing fetal monitors, collecting her pee, and starting an IV. If she met the criteria to be admitted and her cervix wasn't changing 1cm per 1-2 hours, she was getting Pitocin (contraction juice). No questions asked. Epidurals were encouraged, as it was much easier to monitor the baby while the woman was lying comfortably.

Doulas, alternative laboring positions, and natural birth were scoffed at. This was a baby factory, and we knew how to minimize risk and increase the odds of a safe delivery. I owe a world of gratitude to the amazing team of nurses, residents, attendings, and patients who taught me the fundamentals of labor and delivery.

Fast forward a year later. I was newly engaged and about to relocate to Minnesota. I found no labor and delivery jobs posted online, so I reached out to an acquaintance I knew who worked as an OB nurse near the Twin Cities. I had hit pay dirt and accepted a labor and delivery nurse position at Woodwinds in Woodbury, Minnesota.

Five minutes into orientation, it was apparent I was in a completely different world. "What do you mean we don't get baseline blood work on everyone?" I remember asking. Woodwinds was proud of their essential oils, water-births, nature sounds channel, massage, an array of birthing balls, and diversity of providers. The environment was incredibly warm and welcoming. I had no idea a hospital could feel like that.

Initially, I avoided the midwife and hopeful water-birth patients like the plague. I was quick to ask my co-workers to switch assignments with me if I was assigned either. I was intimidated by natural birth and clueless as to how to support an unmedicated woman in labor. Epidurals and a controlled environment defined my comfort zone. I had no plans of opening my mind to a natural birth. It wasn't until I had my own disappointing epidural experience when my first son was born that my mindset began to change.

I had been a labor nurse for two years before I would become the birthing patient. I went into that experience (on the other side of the table!) knowing exactly how my birth was going to go. I would arrive at the hospital in early labor (when I was still smiling and could answer the admission questions with ease.) If my cervix wasn't dilating, I would ask my doctor to break my water and start a "whiff" of Pitocin. I would seize the epidural at the first and slightest sign of discomfort and take a nap while my body would finish dilating and labor down. Of course I would be a great pusher, as I had helped coach countless women to do before! And my baby would be effortlessly welcomed into the world.

The plan was working smoothly until it was clear that my epidural was "one-sided." This happens sometimes. To other women. But I never considered it would happen to me. There was only one anesthesiologist on duty that night, and there was nobody else to attempt a better-centered epidural for full relief. The rest of my labor was a rather "spiritual" experience. I vividly recall being so unprepared for the contractions, the pressure, and the infamous, dreaded "ring of fire." I pushed for two and a half hours, and my bladder has never been the same since! It was after this experience and an unanticipated feeling of disappointment in my labor performance, that I knew there had to be a better way.

A couple of months after my maternity leave, I registered for the Birth Support class offered by Woodwinds. The class was designed to help educate labor and delivery nurses about natural labor and how we could better support our patients. It covered hormones at play, labor techniques, birthing positions and the possible unintended effects of our well-meaning interventions. I was mesmerized. I felt like someone had given me a brand new set of eyes.

From that class forward, I was a different nurse. I found myself hoping to be assigned a patient who wanted to labor without medication. Suddenly, I saw the beauty and advantages of natural births. I stopped over-analyzing the fetal and contraction patterns and began taking care of my patients. I suddenly understood that I could affect how my patients remembered their birth stories, and I wanted a happy and empowering memory for each.

When my second son was born, I prepared for a natural birth and couldn't have been more satisfied. I read up on hypnobirthing and midwife techniques, and I read anti-fear labor books. This time, I trusted my body and didn't depend on the drugs that may or may not be available to me.

I wish every woman would have the tools to take control of her body and her birth. I do believe that epidurals have their place, and I have seen many women successfully have a vaginal birth because of the relaxing properties of an epidural. I have also seen the many benefits of intervention-free births. It is such a privilege to live in a society where women have access to a spectrum of birthing facilities, methods, providers, and techniques.

It is my hope that after reading this book, each expectant mama may recognize the inherent beauty in her body. I also hope she will realize she can trust it (along with helpful tools) to be prepared for labor and birth. I hope to instill confidence in the amazing nurses and providers serving our communities and to dispel the myth that hospitals are a scary place where births are manipulated to ensure your provider is home in time for dinner. Your nurses, providers and I want your birth story to be a happy one.

Chapter One
You Have Options

"There is a secret in our culture, and it's not that birth is painful. It's that women are strong."

--Laura Stavoe Harm

Congratulations! The test was positive, and you're pregnant. Your first decision is likely how to share the news with your partner and maybe a few close loved ones. You may be beginning to feel the early signs of pregnancy, as nausea and constipation settle in. Welcome to the club! Sooner or later, it's time to schedule your first appointment, and you may be overwhelmed by not knowing whom to call. You may call your insurance carrier for in-network providers or begin looking up reviews of medical professionals in your area.

Before selecting the provider who's right for you, you should know the differences between the primary categories of providers: family practice doctor, Certified Nurse Midwife, Licensed Homebirth Midwife, and OB/GYN.

Family practice doctors appeal to those who value continuity of care. She has been your go-to gal for everything from the stomach flu to your first pap-smear. She has been with you through it all, and you trust her. If you are relatively healthy and your family practice doctor delivers babies (not all do), this may be a great option for you. Another benefit to a family practice doctor is that s/he will take care of your baby after birth as well. A family practice doctor is the only provider option that offers both prenatal and newborn care. A family practice doctor may not be for you if you want a birth specialist who can handle the full scope of labor through delivery. Family practice doctors do not perform cesarean births, and if complications or concerns arise in pregnancy or labor, an OB/GYN will be consulted and may take over your care. If considering a family practice doctor for your prenatal care, it is important to interview him/her and ask how many births s/he has attended in the past year. You should also ask about the parameters of conditions that would prompt a family practice doctor to potentially transfer your care to an OB/GYN.

Midwives are another great option for low-risk pregnancies and healthy mamas. Midwives specialize in women's health and are amongst the most attentive birth attendants. A majority of midwives have labor nursing backgrounds and dedicate themselves to helping implement your birth plan. Midwives are more likely to accommodate alternative labor techniques, water-births, and flexibility with birthing positions. Certified Nurse Midwives who practice in a hospital setting generally work in groups and are required to have an obstetrician (commonly called an OB/GYN or OB) backup if concerns arise during pregnancy, labor, or delivery.

Similar to family practice doctor limitations, your care may be transferred to the OB/GYN backup at any time if certain complications arise. When interviewing a potential midwife for your care, it's a good idea to ask about the specifics of these parameters. In some states, midwives may legally attend planned home births. Licensed Homebirth Midwives are prevalent in Canada and the United Kingdom.

Lastly, an obstetrician may be an especially great option for you if you have a complicated medical history or want the assurance of knowing your provider won't be handing off care no matter how your birth story unfolds. Much of an obstetrician's education focuses on detecting and managing complications in pregnancy and labor. If you desire a more hands-off or natural approach, it is important to interview a potential OB/GYN about their comfort level and willingness to accommodate your wishes.

Whomever you choose, it is essential to ask where the provider has privileges to deliver. Each hospital or birth center has a list of providers that are approved to deliver at that facility. If you are hoping to deliver at a specific hospital or birth center, ensure your provider has these privileges. With any provider, it is important to reflect on what is most important to you for your baby's delivery and discuss these goals together. Specific goals often vary from individual to individual.

While the provider's responses to your questions are key, the more telling indications about their beliefs and attitudes may be found in their nonverbal cues. Does s/he seem annoyed by your questions? Or is genuine openness relayed? Is there defensiveness in his or her tone or calm openness? Some example discussion guidelines are as follows:

- We are hoping and planning for a natural birth. How will you support us in this goal? (Supportive answers may include intermittent--rather than constant-- monitoring, ability to walk and move around the room or unit, use of tubs and exercise balls during labor, holding off on augmentation measures that may push labor along like breaking the water or starting IV Pitocin.)

- What percent of babies do you deliver by Cesarean? (The national average cesarean rate is around 30% of

9

births; however, there are providers that have a much lower rate, as low 5-10%.)

- What are your feelings towards assertive pushing versus laboring down? (Assertive pushing can be exhausting and sometimes cause unnecessary swelling. Laboring down is gaining popularity as it affords the mother to continue to rest and breathe through her contractions as her body naturally nudges the baby lower in the birth canal cutting down on pushing time. Laboring down is especially beneficial if the mother has an epidural and a decreased urge to push. Often naturally birthing moms have a strong involuntary urge to push and may not find laboring down helpful.

- Do you have specific time limits on labor and/or pushing before intervention? (It is normal for first time mothers to be completely dilated and pushing for 2-4 hours prior to delivery; however, some providers are more lenient with a little extra time if progress is being made.)

Selecting a facility that will accommodate your birthing hopes can be just as important as picking a provider. Not all hospitals are created equal. Each facility has a rating and corresponding level of care regarding its ability to care for the newborn.

Level 3 hospitals can provide all services including NICU (Neonatal Intensive Care Unit) for critically ill newborns. Level 2 hospitals generally have a skilled nursery for stable babies needing some intervention. Level 1 hospitals provide basic care.

If delivering at either a Level 2 or Level 1 facility, it is possible that the baby would need to be transferred, usually via ambulance, to a Level 3 facility. Some healthy moms with low-risk pregnancies choose to deliver at Level 3 hospitals for the peace of mind they offer. If unexpected complications arise, the mom has added assurance that her baby will have access to the most immediate and skilled care available. This will help ensure that her baby will not be transferred to a separate facility.

It is a good idea to tour potential facilities early in your pregnancy while searching for the best match of both provider and what feels like a safe environment for your birth. A list of suggested questions for your tour follows, but again, it is best to reflect on what is most important to you and ask questions accordingly.

- Would I be allowed to walk around on and/or off of the labor unit after being admitted? (Movement during labor is essential for the baby to be able to rotate as needed prior to delivery. The baby's specific positioning can be essential for a quick and more comfortable birth experience. If a baby gets "stuck" in an unfavorable position, the labor and birth may be lengthened by hours and sometimes may lead to cesarean birth.)

- What natural birthing tools are available on the floor (i.e. birthing balls, birthing stools, squat bars, etc.)? (It is important to find tools that work for you. Even if walking is your plan for movement, you will need to rest and may want a change of pace. Birthing balls are great to set beside a slightly elevated bed. This allows you to rest your upper body on a pillow while slowly circling your hips for comfort. Squatting bars are sometimes used with longer pushing lengths to offer a more upright way to birth your baby.)

- Are the nurses specifically trained in supporting natural labor? (This was a game-changer for me as a nurse. Prior to the training, I didn't understand how to best support a natural laboring mother. This training gave me wonderful tools to be able to suggest as well as motivated me to advocate for my patients' birth plans.)

- Are tubs available during labor? (Water is naturally relaxing as well as helps to make the contractions feel shorter. Another benefit is it is often easier to change positions in a tub rather than laying in a bed. Moms often find tubs help to make the labor more comfortable.)

- Is this a baby-friendly facility? (Baby-friendly is an initiative designed especially to support breastfeeding mothers.)

- Are statistics on inductions, epidurals, and cesarean births available? (Higher rates of these categories may indicate that the staff is not well informed about natural birth techniques and may not offer to help support your goals.)

• What are your policies on eating and drinking during labor? (It is standard to not be able to eat after having an epidural placed as this is an anesthesia rule; however, some facilities and/or providers also may restrict women without an epidural. As laboring takes a considerable amount of energy, it's important that you are able to be well nourished and hydrated.)

Chapter Two
What to Expect During Pregnancy

"Instead of wishing away nine months of pregnancy complaining about the shadow over my feet, I'd have cherished every minute of it and realized that the wonderment growing inside me was to be my only chance in life to assist God in a miracle."

--Erma Bombeck

The first trimester. Perhaps Charles Dickens captured the first three months of pregnancy best with "It was the best of times, it was the worst of times."[1] The thrill of the first faint positive test is a special kind of high for many expecting mamas. Often, a baby has been longed for and prayed for. For couples actively trying to conceive, waiting to test is like the long, slow seemingly endless climb to the top of a rollercoaster. The positive test then is like the tip top rush where you peak over the edge and let yourself fall.

Conversely, not all pregnancies are necessarily convenient or expected. In these cases, the positive test may feel less like a rush and more like a nauseating plunge. Wherever you are on this rollercoaster, know that you are not alone and however you feel is absolutely okay.

Hormones, hormones, hormones. They'll make you want to sleep for days. They'll make your boobs ache. They'll make you, oh, so queasy and may just make you lose your breakfast, lunch, and/or dinner. If the nausea wasn't unsettling enough, often women have a heightened sense of smell in those early weeks. Fantastic! During my first pregnancy in particular, I worked nights, and my husband would get ready for work shortly after I fell asleep in the morning. I would wake up a few hours later and could still catch whiffs of his hairspray. That faint lingering scent would promptly send me to the toilet retching. I wanted to kill him. How inconsiderate, right? Did I mention hormonal mood swings? Ha! But seriously, a heightened sense of smell, food aversions, food cravings, extreme exhaustion, acne, a rollercoaster of emotion, and last - but most certainly not least irritating- constipation are all very common. Especially in the beginning of pregnancy.

Anxiety and over-analyzing every cramp, gas bubble, and twinge is also very common as your Mama Bear mode kicks in. What's important to keep in mind is that there is a very wide range of normal symptoms during all of pregnancy.

There are a few concerning parameters to watch for, but overall, most changes are perfectly within the realm of normal. Mild cramping and even a little bit of spotting or light bleeding can be normal. With any bleeding, it is important to wear a pad to help quantify how much bleeding you are experiencing. Your provider will want to know this information.

Normal causes of bleeding include implantation (generally occurs about 10 days after ovulation around day 22-25 of cycle and is pink and light in nature prior to a positive pregnancy test) and commonly a subchorionic hemorrhage (a small pocket of blood between the uterine wall and the amniotic sac that generally resolves). Even though light bleeding or spotting most often resolves without medical intervention, you should always contact your provider to report bleeding during pregnancy. Other symptoms to always report are: severe abdominal or pelvic pain, sharp pain just under the right breast (called epigastric pain which could indicate need for further labs and monitoring), altered vision, and persistent or worsening headaches.

As your pregnancy progresses, the nausea and fatigue will likely subside and be replaced by an ever-growing bump that brings along a new set of aches and pains for some women. These aches and pains are usually normal and are most likely caused by your muscles stretching to accommodate your growing baby and bag of water.

Some women experience intense heartburn, sciatic or round ligament pain, and even pregnancy-induced carpal tunnel in their hands and wrists. Unfortunately, some of these pains may persist until the baby is born. The good news is even these miserable discomforts are not worrisome as far as the health of your baby is concerned. Comfort measures include: staying hydrated by drinking several glasses of water a day, warm baths, positioning with pillows, supportive belts or braces, balancing rest and activity, and TYLENOL® as directed on bottle. You should contact your provider to report persistent or worsening pain.

As you can see, there are plenty of not-so-glamorous aspects to being pregnant. And yet, pregnant women are often described as having that "radiant glow." This is a season that you have license to slow down and focus on caring for yourself and your growing baby. Relish in the magnificent work your body is instinctively carrying out. It is truly phenomenal.

Another remarkable phenomenon common in pregnancy are vivid - and often very strange - dreams. A cousin of mine reported dreaming that she caught her very straight farmer-husband having an affair with another man. I had a vivid dream about giving birth at home and upon nursing my precious baby, I realized my breast had morphed into the face of an opossum! I later googled "dreaming about an opossum" and was surprised to discover that opossums often appear in dreams when an individual is nervous or anxious about something, commonly about motherhood. Outrageous, I know!

Another time my husband woke me up as he thought I was having difficulty breathing. Apparently, I was panting as if I was doing one hundred jumping jacks. Turns out, I was dreaming that I was horseback herding cattle across France! I can still close my eyes and see the dust surrounding me and hear the sound of thousands of stampeding hooves in my ears. This dream was intense! I remember being so annoyed that he woke me up from my epic adventure.

This is a good place to pause and mention that even though vivid dreams to this degree were unusual for me, I was able to discern the difference between unusual and concerning. Although, I typically don't dream about parts of my body morphing into a rodent or experience the rush of horseback riding, I didn't need to consult my doctor about my unusual dreams. In our well-meaning but often overly anxious and analytical states, sometimes it seems that we need to report every little unexpected thing. Although, it's good to pay attention and listen to our bodies, obsessing over the small stuff only reinforces a mindset of panic and worry. It can be detrimental to a peaceful and joyful birth experience.

Towards the last few weeks of pregnancy, Braxton Hicks contractions (a tightening sensation in your abdomen) often summon your inner detective to report for duty as you return to your over-analyzing ways. Frequently, the uterus begins to flex its muscle in preparation for labor. This can be very frustrating, as contractions may be consistent for hours and then suddenly stop. Or the contractions can just keep you uncomfortable enough where it is impossible to think of anything else. Before you go to your provider to be evaluated, I recommend drinking a large glass of water and taking a warm shower or bath to help rule out or rule in labor. If rhythmic tightening persists after these measures and continues to become stronger and closer together, you should contact your provider.

Spotting or light bleeding can also appear at the end of pregnancy as your cervix softens, thins, and even begins to dilate. While we're on the topic of normal spotting, let's just talk about the infamous mucus plug for a minute, can we? First of all, gross. It's often a thick, blood-streaked jelly-like substance that dislodges from the cervix at some point prior to labor. Precious, right? This may seem like a significant event, but it actually gives zero information about how soon your baby will be born. Sometimes the plug makes an appearance on the day of delivery, but it also may appear a couple of weeks ahead of your baby's birthday. Some women don't notice losing this plug at all. It truly is irrelevant and its appearance absolutely doesn't mean that you are in labor. The great news is you are free to stop investigating your toilet paper!

Eventually, the final weeks of your pregnancy will arrive, and it may just feel like time comes to a halt. The last couple of weeks can be the slowest, as you feel the baby could come at any time. Your impending labor is likely the only thing you can think about as you perpetually prepare for your baby's arrival. Sleep notoriously becomes more and more interrupted. Putting on your socks and shaving your legs may seem like overwhelming and cruel tasks. Hang in there, mama. You will not be pregnant forever, and these discomforts somehow make meeting your baby all the more joyous.

Chapter Three
Prepare Your Body, Mind, and Spirit

"Within you there is a stillness and a

sanctuary to which you can retreat at any time."

--Herman Hesse

The body, mind, and spirit work best when integrated, working in harmony with each other. Integrity means being whole. Undivided. Athletes know this. Mental preparation, relaxation, and visualization techniques are arguably just as important as their physical preparation.

Within us, there is a storehouse of confidence, calmness, and power that we can tap into at any time. Our bodies often carry out actions that begin in our mind. We must first believe we are able to do something before we put our bodies in motion to carry it out. Achieving this integrity between mind, body, and spirit is the goal for an empowering, calm and satisfying pregnancy and birth.

Our bodies are incredible and accomplish astonishing things intuitively. It truly is fascinating. Did you know that the average person takes 23,000 breaths per day without ever thinking about it? The average heart beats 115,000 times per day. All that is required on our part to keep this machine running smoothly are good fuel and a bit of exercise.

One of the easiest and most essential ways to maintain a healthy body and a healthy pregnancy is to make sure you are drinking enough water. (The standard recommendation of "enough" is at least 64 ounces, and the more optimal goal is 96 ounces). Dehydration in pregnancy often leads to dizziness, headaches, decreased fetal movement, and even uterine irritability (cramping). Not only is sufficient water consumption vital for the significant increase in blood volume during pregnancy, but it is helpful in avoiding common discomforts and complications like cramping, constipation and joint pain.

Along with staying well hydrated, proper nutrition is key to your baby's wellbeing. Pregnancy is a great time to make a new resolution to eating well if you haven't had healthy habits in the past. You are your baby's only source of nutrition, so what you put in your mouth should be taken seriously. You should discuss your diet with your provider for the most up-to-date recommendations and a list of foods to avoid.

It is most beneficial to consume a variety of foods to ensure the array of nutrients needed to support your baby's development. The American Congress of Obstetricians and Gynecologists (ACOG) [2] recommends making one half of your plate fruits and vegetables to ensure adequate vitamins and minerals to support your growing baby. On average, only an extra 300 "well-chosen" calories should be consumed per day to support your pregnancy and an 600 extra calories if you are carrying twins. These recommendations are intended for women within the normal range for body mass index (BMI). You can calculate your BMI using an online calculator like the following: www.nhlbi.nih.gov/health/educational/lose_wt/BMI/.

Another important key to physical health in pregnancy is exercise. It is generally advised that you may continue your pre-pregnancy workout regimens. If you were physically active before getting pregnant, it is usually safe to continue the same activities. It is important to listen to your body and take breaks when needed. If you were not physically active prior to pregnancy but are hoping to initiate exercise, some safe beginner suggestions include: walking, swimming, low-impact aerobics, and indoor stationary cycling.

I recommend yoga for anyone but especially for expecting mamas. Of the hundreds of births I've witnessed, yogi moms tend to experience the easiest and calmest ones. Yoga is low impact and supports a healthy core while gradually stretching muscles to promote flexibility. A strong core, flexibility, and breathing techniques that come from intentional practice will absolutely be your friends in labor. If you are interested in practicing yoga but are not necessarily ready to sign up for a class, there is a world of free beginner classes available on YouTube.

It is good to set realistic fitness goals for yourself. A realistic goal can be as simple as doing yoga 3 times per week for 20 minutes. Statistics show that people are more likely to achieve their goals if they are written down, challenging but not overwhelming, and measurable. You should discuss exercise regimens with your provider prior to starting something new and if any concerns should arise related to a specific activity.

Now that you have your physical health covered, let's dig a little deeper. Disciplining the mind is one of the most powerful gifts you can give yourself. Martin Luther wisely observed, "You cannot keep birds from flying over your head but you can keep them from building a nest in your hair."[3] Although you may not have control over every thought or fear that creeps into your mind, you can absolutely decide what thoughts you feed and give life to.

Cultivating practices of intentional gratitude and optimism can empower you to focus on the good and to let go of what you cannot control. Disciplining the mind enables you to conquer fears and anxieties, which is essential in achieving a calm pregnancy and birth.

Effectively conditioning the mind for ultimate relaxation does take intentional daily practice. Marie Mongan writes in her book HypnoBirthing The Mongan Method, "While birthing should not be the exhausting, pushing-your-body-to-the-edge feat that athletes face, it nevertheless requires the same kind of discipline so that when the time comes, you are ready. Since you are conditioning your mind for ultimate relaxation, it is important that you form a pattern that your mind can automatically respond to when it comes time for your birthing. It is time well spent, and it can cut the time and the effort you will spend in your labor. As one who has been there, I can emphatically say that conditioning is a must. You can't slough it off and hope that you'll get lucky."[4]

If you haven't already established an intentional breathing and relaxation practice, here are some tips to get started. First, it's important to carve out at least 10 to 20 minutes every day that you can be quiet and still. If you can spare longer, even better. This time should be a priority - but not a chore. This should be a happy place and something you look forward to.

Next, you'll want to find an environment that is calm, quiet, and comfortable. Your bed may be an excellent choice as it's already deeply associated with safety and relaxation. Soft music, nature sounds, or even playing the HypnoBirthing CD (which can be found at www.hypnobirthing.com) will help guide your body into a deep state of relaxation. Lastly, get into a comfortable position, close your eyes, breathe, and visualize.

For the first couple of minutes, it's a good practice to focus solely on your breathing. Try to slow your breathing and intentionally expand your breathing capacity. An effective technique to do this is to softly close your eyes while you practice counting with your own inhalations and exhalations. As you inhale, gradually and steadily count in your head from one to five. Then pause, and count as you exhale from one to five. Try to gradually increase your ending number by one with each inhalation and exhalation. So as you inhale with your next breath, count from one to six, and so on. I love how simple and effective this technique is. It is a great technique to draw from during labor, as it helps to instill that each contraction will eventually end. Your only - and so doable - job is to keep breathing.

Wonderful breathing techniques can be found online and in several labor books. I highly recommend HypnoBirthing The Mongan Method, as a great guide with wonderful tools to help achieve a calm and more comfortable birth experience.

If the HypnoBirthing method seems too much for you or you are skeptical of hypno-anything, I get it. I was raised Evangelical Christian, and had only negative associations with any kind of hypnotism, meditation, and any spiritual work that didn't explicitly come from the bible or from the church. I was taught that these spiritual practices and notions were somehow dangerous and even evil. As an adult, I have reconsidered my beliefs and now see God working through these practices. Much like I see eating an orange as a gift that comes from God, even though the sticker suggests I should give the credit to Sunkist.

The realization that some of the most beautiful births I had seen used hypnobirthing techniques (whether the mother realized it or not) and overhearing one of my patient's hypnobirthing CDs in labor helped me to realize that there is nothing remotely satanic or evil about it. Through these births I had witnessed and even in my own birth experience, I came to understand that it is possible to achieve a state of calmness while also being fully present. Even though I had come to believe that I wouldn't be going against God in using hypnobirth techniques, I was concerned that the techniques might put me in a daze of sorts. I feared I might somehow lose being consciously present because of the hypnosis aspect.

The term hypnosis is defined as "the induction of a state of consciousness in which a person apparently loses the power of voluntary action and is highly responsive to suggestion or direction." Losing "power of voluntary action" is what I didn't want to experience. The goal of these techniques for me and I believe for most women who are interested in using them is to have a sense of empowerment - not loss of power. I am so grateful that I was able to witness this empowerment firsthand! I'm grateful too that I was able to see past what I believe to be the misleading and unfortunate naming of these invaluable birthing techniques.

Still not for you? That's absolutely ok. The beautiful thing about birthing techniques is that you get to pick and choose what resonates and what would be helpful to you personally. Guided visualization is another wonderful technique that you may find helpful. I recommend having fun creating your own sanctuary in your mind. I love to search pictures online of beautiful destinations for inspiration and then visualize myself in that environment. As I'm personally drawn to beautiful beaches, I like to close my eyes and try to feel the sand between my toes and the sun on my shoulders. I picture myself being calm and happy, as I take in the most gorgeous view. I can escape to this world of lakes (without mosquitos) and oceans (without the threat of shark attacks) any time I like.

The fun part about your personal paradise is that it can be as detailed or as simple as you like. It truly is whatever you want it to be, and you can change it up as you like. Maybe for you a specific visualization is helpful in achieving a deep sense of calm. You may want to return to the same place again and again. You may find a sense of happy relaxation for a while in returning to the same space, but over time it may become boring or dull. It is absolutely okay to completely change everything about this happy place. Some days you may be in the mood for a tropical paradise, and other days call for a cozy spot high on snow-capped mountains. Our minds are truly amazing things, and I hope that you fall in love with this new practice of retreating to your inner sanctuary.

The final component of our journey to being healthy, whole, and integrated is the spirit. Rea Nolan Martin writes in her article "How to Feed the Body, Mind, and Spirit" published by the Huffington Post:

> "Most of us understand the spirit in the context of religion, but modern scientific study of energy has brought new meaning to the term. In these circles, the words "spiritual" and "energetic" are often used interchangeably. This is because the spirit is no longer viewed as an abstract entity, but as a distinctive vibrational field--the actual energetic host of your mind and body.
>
> Our spirits are the most intimate things about us, and ironically, the least familiar. No matter your context or definition, the means of nourishing the spirit is the same.
>
> 1. Pray—You are never really powerless when prayer is sincerely invoked. It's a means of letting go, acknowledging God, and releasing your praise or problems to the casual level where wholeness (and solutions) exist. Reactive prayer is a good beginning - as long as it's affirmative. Recite a prayer or create your own. Prayer works. By releasing the ego, the spirit becomes expansive, allowing change to occur.
> 2. Meditate—This time I'm suggesting a deeper practice called contemplation. Sit quietly and concentrate on your breathing. In and out. Clear your screen--no words, images, or concepts. You are intentionally

placing yourself in the divine presence. So be alert. Maybe not this time, or next time, but with deliberation and purity of intention, at some point, you will experience a greater connection to the Source. In addition to the spiritual benefits, there are countless mental and physical benefits to this practice, including deep peace and healing on a cellular level. Combine it with breathing exercise, and start with ten minutes. It's worth the time.

3. Participate—Prayerful communal ritual elevates the spirit. Participating in a compassionate community that serves others will bless you too. With respect to preaching, keep in mind the words of St. Francis: "Preach the Gospel; use words only when necessary." Preach by example and with humility always. There is more we don't know than we do."[5]

Spirituality is the essence and energy we radiate to ourselves and everyone around us. As mentioned above, the greatest thing we can do for our own spiritual health is to maintain a high level of humility and willingness to let go of control. This is a very difficult thing to put into practice for most of us, but there is a profound sense of freedom if we will allow ourselves to surrender and acknowledge that much of life is beyond our control. Here's to strong, happy, healthy, and beautiful bodies, minds, and souls.

Chapter Four
Birth Plan

"Don't just wish for a great birth, prepare for one."

--Birthbootcamp.com

If a happy and deeply satisfying birth story is your goal, then it is essential to reflect on exactly what that statement uniquely means to you. Some women may find importance in a calm and intimate environment via soft lighting or music. Others may want intermittent, rather than constant, fetal monitoring and the luxury of being able to labor with the freedoms they choose (such as being able to eat once admitted). Many labor and delivery units have policies and protocols that may or may not accommodate a mother's specific wishes. However, many wishes on a typical birth plan are standard in many hospitals and birth centers (such as skin-to-skin time immediately following the birth). Discussing your birth plan with your provider and/or bringing it with you to a hospital or birth center tour may help to give you a sense of what on your list is easy to accommodate (or even standard) and what wishes may not be as easily served.

It may be helpful to think of your birth plan more in terms of birth preferences, as the term plan may be perceived by the staff as a rigid list of demands. It is beneficial to acknowledge and come to terms with the fact that there are many variables within each birth story that are out of your provider's and your own control. An example of this would be the development of a fever in labor. Nobody plans on this scenario, but it happens commonly. If untreated with TYLENOL®, antibiotics and fluids, the baby's heart rate will more than likely become elevated (tachycardic). If you are flexible enough to listen to your provider and discuss risks and benefits of interventions in the moment, the fever may be resolved quickly and nothing more than just a small bump in the road. However, if you are holding tightly to an intervention-free labor and birth plan and refuse any intervention for any reason, it could be detrimental to your natural birth wishes. Detrimental as in prolonged fetal tachycardia may move to prolonged decelerations and can often result in an emergent cesarean section.

Chances are your labor will be complication-free. After all, humans have been giving birth for thousands of years prior to modern monitoring and interventions. However, sometimes big or small unforeseen complications occur, and it's good to have an openness towards letting details of your plan go for the ultimate goal of a healthy baby.

To create your birth plan or list of birth preferences, I suggest dreaming about your ideal labor and birth. Make note of what the room looks like. Are you laboring in a bathtub or swaying with your partner beside the bed? What are you wearing? Is a hospital gown acceptable to you? Or would you rather wear your own sports bra or robe if possible? What interventions are you open to? After the baby is born, what expectations do you have? Documenting these hopes and highlighting your top two to three priorities is a wonderful tool to help you achieve a happy birth memory.

Example birth plan modified from:
https://www.thebump.com/a/tool-birth-plan

[ ] Name and Partner's name:

[ ] Due date (or induction date):

[ ] Provider's name:

My delivery is anticipated to be:

[ ] Vaginal

[ ] Water birth

[ ] Caesarean Section

I'd like _____ present before AND/OR during labor:

[ ] Partner:

[ ] Other children:

[ ] Other:

During labor, I'd like:

[ ] Music played (I will provide)

[ ] The lights dimmed

[ ] The room as quiet as possible

[ ] As few interruptions as possible

[ ] As few vaginal exams as possible

[ ] Hospital staff limited to my own doctor and nurses (no students, residents or interns present)

[ ] To be assigned a nurse who is partial to natural birthing

[ ] To wear my own clothes

[ ] My partner to film AND/OR take pictures

[ ] My partner to be present the entire time

[ ] To stay hydrated with clear liquids and ice chips

[ ] To eat and drink as approved by my doctor

I'd like fetal monitoring to be:

[ ] Continuous

[ ] Internal only if deemed necessary

[ ] Performed only by Doppler

[ ] Intermittent

[ ] External only

I'd like labor augmentation:

[ ] Performed only if baby is in distress

[ ] First attempted by natural methods

[ ] Performed with Pitocin

[ ] Performed by rupture of the membrane

[ ] Never to include an artificial rupture of the membrane

For pain relief, I'd like to use:

[ ] Acupressure if available

[ ] Breathing techniques

[ ] Intravenous (IV) medication

[ ] Massage

[ ] Nitrous Oxide gas if available

[ ] Epidural

[ ] Hypnobirth techniques

[ ] Meditation

As the baby is delivered, I would like to:

[ ] Push spontaneously

[ ] Push as directed

[ ] Push without time limits, as long as the baby and I are not at risk

[ ] Use a mirror to see the baby crown

[ ] Let the epidural wear off while pushing

[ ] Have a full dose of epidural

[ ] Avoid vacuum extraction

[ ] Open to discuss methods my doctor recommends or deems necessary

[ ] Help catch the baby

[ ] Let my partner catch the baby

I would like an episiotomy:

[ ] Used only after perineal massage, warm compresses and positioning

[ ] Rather than risk a tear

[ ] Not performed, even if it means risking a tear

[ ] Performed only as a last resort as my provider deems necessary

[ ] Performed with local anesthesia

Immediately after delivery, I would like:

[ ] My partner to cut the umbilical cord

[ ] To bank the cord blood

[ ] To donate the cord blood

[ ] Not to be given Pitocin/oxytocin

[ ] To deliver the placenta spontaneously and without assistance

[ ] To see the placenta before it is discarded

[ ] The umbilical cord to be cut only after it stops pulsating

If a C-section is necessary, I would like:

[ ] To make sure all other options have been exhausted

[ ] My partner to remain with me the entire time

[ ] The screen lowered so I can watch baby come out

[ ] My hands left free so I can touch the baby

[ ] My partner to hold the baby as soon as possible

[ ] To be assisted in skin-to-skin time as soon as possible

I would like to hold baby:

[ ] Immediately after delivery

[ ] After baby is dried and swaddled

[ ] Before eye drops/ointment are given

I would like to breastfeed:

[ ] As soon as possible after delivery

[ ] Before eye drops/ointment are given

[ ] Within an hour of delivery

[ ] Not interested

I'd like baby's medical exam, bath, and procedures:

[ ] Given in my presence

[ ] Given only after we've bonded

[ ] To include a hearing screening test

[ ] To include a heel stick for screening tests beyond the PKU

[ ] To include a hepatitis B vaccine

Please don't give baby:

[ ] Vitamin K

[ ] Antibiotic eye treatment

[ ] Sugar water

[ ] Formula

[ ] A pacifier

I'd like to feed baby:

[ ] Only with breastmilk

[ ] Only with formula

[ ] May supplement breastfeeding with formula

If we have a boy, circumcision should:

[ ] Be performed

[ ] Not be performed

[ ] Be performed after discharge in the clinic

[ ] Be performed in the presence of me AND/OR my partner

As needed post-delivery, please give me:

[ ] Extra-strength acetaminophen

[ ] Percocet

[ ] Ibuprofen

[ ] Stool softener

If baby is not well, I'd like:

[ ] My partner and I to accompany it to the NICU or another facility

[ ] To breastfeed or provide pumped breastmilk

[ ] To hold him or her whenever possible

Example birth plan for the more 'go with the flow' planners among us:

1. Trust my provider's and nurse's recommendations
2. Have baby
3. Try not to swear
4. Eat celebratory Chipotle burrito

No matter if you are a detailed planner or are happy with your birth center's standards of care, making a list of your top priorities or goals will help your providers, nurses, and loved ones know how to support you in writing your beautiful birth story.

Chapter Five Labor
Let Your Monkey Do It

"The mind is the perceptor and interpreter of stimuli; it is in the mind that pain in normal labour arises. The best and safest anaesthetic is an educated and controlled mind."

Grantly Dick-Read, Childbirth Without Fear

Most of us are conditioned to fear, to some degree, the pain of childbirth. Maybe your well-intentioned mother or school sex educator used fear of pregnancy and the pain of childbirth as a tactic to get you to abstain in high school. Movie scenes and TV shows generally depict labor and birth in a dramatic and often alarming light. Also, our culture seems to value one-upping each other in storytelling. This has influenced the tendency of women we know to brag about their labor suffering to elicit sympathy or at least impress their listener. The worst stories are those that get shared most often and deeply inflict a level of anxiety or fear towards childbirth, even subconsciously.

Unfortunately, most women have heard less-than-pleasant birth stories and approach labor as something to suffer through or possibly avoid all together. Labor becomes something we approach with fear and timidity, than than approaching it with confidence that our bodies are strong and made for this. Our bodies know exactly what they're doing. Many women who fear labor decide before ever feeling their first contraction that they will request an epidural as soon as possible to avoid the anticipated suffering.

I was one of these women as I approached the birth of my first son. I understand the fear of extreme vulnerability. There is the vulnerability of laboring in front of loved ones. And, because I delivered both my boys on the labor and delivery unit I worked on, I also experienced the vulnerability of laboring in full view of my coworkers. I definitely didn't want to be a screamer or awful and rude. I knew that labor could bring about a woman's rawness, and I wasn't sure I wanted to be so exposed. Even though I had seen several beautiful and calm births, I had also seen many not-so-serene ones. I didn't know then that a calm birth is something that can be prepared for. I assumed the women who experienced calm births just got lucky.

Back then at a very deep level, I saw the vulnerability and pain of labor as something to fear. So I concluded that getting an epidural early in active labor would afford me a good nap prior to pushing, and I would painlessly birth my baby. This works for a lot of women, and I had seen it work. I believe that epidurals can be effective in helping mothers achieve a state of deep relaxation, especially in our anxiety-prone culture. I didn't expect that my epidural would be one-sided (sometimes epidurals are malpositioned when placed. They may initially achieve a sense of numbness throughout the abdominal area and legs, but after the initial bolus dose wears off, pain or feeling returns to the left or right side of the abdomen and pelvic region. If this occurs, your nurse should call anesthesia to adjust the line or even replace it; however, sometimes, adequate coverage isn't achieved despite their efforts to "fix" it.) I also didn't expect that I would actually have to do and feel the work of labor.

Had everything gone according to my plan, I may never have fallen in love with natural birth. In the weeks and months following my first son's birth, I had an undeniable feeling of disappointment about how my labor went. It's difficult to put into words the complexity of this feeling. I knew that I wanted to give labor and birth another shot, but, the next time, I wanted to feel strong and united with my body rather than powerless.

Coincidentally, a couple of months after I returned from maternity leave, I was due to take a Labor Support class through my employer. Little did I know that the information I would receive in that class would forever transform my view of birth.

I remember being completely fascinated as my coworker explained the intricate dance between hormones, anatomy, and environment that have significant influence on how labor plays out. I was captivated by the natural hormones at play and how truly amazing and capable our bodies are. Of course I knew about oxytocin "contraction juice" and vaguely recalled that prolactin had something to do with breastfeeding.

However, most of my labor training revolved around keeping mom and baby safe. This meant learning and carrying out protocols and providers' orders (everything from how often to take the mother's blood pressure to when to call the provider for delivery). The most important protocol was analyzing contraction and fetal heart rate patterns.

Prior to this class, I had been a labor nurse for about three years. Until then, no one had ever explained in detail the fundamental biology our bodies instinctively follow. Even if science is low on the list of your interests, I encourage you to give the following description of hormones some thought. Hopefully, you will see the wonder and genius of your body. Ideally, you'll learn to trust it. I believe that your understanding of the natural hormones in labor and birth is a game-changer because you'll better understand the disruptive role of anxiety and fear in the labor process. You'll also begin to understand and trust that you were made for this.

Natural Labor Hormones

- **Prolactin**
  - Peaks at birth
  - Responsible for milk production
  - Induces maternal behavior
  - Complements Oxytocin
- **Oxytocin (The love hormone)**
  - Rhythmic release is responsible for uterine contractions
  - Enables bonding between mother and baby
  - High levels provide feeling of euphoria at birth
  - Helps in birthing placenta
  - Helps control postpartum bleeding and prevents hemorrhage following birth
  - Responsible for milk ejection reflex
  - Inhibited by adrenaline
- **Endorphins**
  - Natural pain relief produced by our bodies
  - Reduces effects of stress
  - Induces feelings of pleasure and euphoria
  - Stimulated by light massage, touch, and laughter
  - Facilitates release of prolactin
  - Elevated levels after birth support mother-baby bonding
- **Melatonin**

- Released in dark quiet settings
- Inhibited by interruption and observation
- Boosts oxytocin
- **Adrenaline**
  - Released under anxiety, fear, and stress
  - Increases heart and breathing rates in mother which lead to elevated heart rate in fetus
  - Slows and blocks oxytocin which inhibits uterine contractions especially in early labor.
  - Associated with prolonged and dysfunctional labor

When I look at how these hormones naturally interact, I'm filled with wonder at what our bodies were made to do. Women instinctively know how to give birth, but our minds and the fears that we've absorbed up to this point intimidate us. The truth is our bodies know how to give birth just like they know how to breathe.

I think it's funny and perhaps helpful to consider the irony in how easy it is to accept that animals instinctively know how to give birth. I'm talking every species from fish laying eggs to elephants. I'm not sure when I started entertaining the idea that the human race was any different. This instinctual birthing ability across all living things dispels fear in me. I hope it does the same for you.

In her blog, Lindsey Welch does a wonderful job articulating the birth experience and the hormones at work,

"Women instinctively know how to give birth. If you give them the space, support and safety they require, women instinctively know what to do when the time comes. The cat silently moves to a dark corner of the room and waits. When everything is quiet and there is nothing to disturb her, she quietly gives birth to her babies. During my Mother's Blessing for my second child, a good friend gave me a stretching cat figurine instead of a traditional bead. "This is to remind you of how cats give birth", she told me, "we can learn a lot from cats". If you look at any creature giving birth in the wild, the same factors apply. Typically nighttime, typically quiet and definitely without disturbance and without being overlooked by others. This is all a world away from the way most women give birth today. If animals need to feel safe and undisturbed in order to labor effectively, then so do humans."[6]

I have observed this "typically nighttime, typically quiet, and definitely without disturbance" phenomenon that Lindsey touches on as a labor nurse. Even if the labor is completed during daytime hours, often the initial wave of contractions begin at night. This makes sense on multiple levels. At a basic hormonal level, we see that Melatonin, our body's sleep hormone, boosts oxytocin, our body's contraction hormone. Also, when our bodies are sleeping, there is absence of anxiety and fear (unless perhaps we're having one of those crazy pregnancy dreams). Achieving sleep also indicates that we are safe, which is another cue to our bodies that it is ok to labor.

This delicate balance of hormones required to labor effectively that Lindsey refers to was the biggest influence on me in desiring birth without an epidural. The medications in the epidural itself didn't concern me as much as the liters of IV fluids that would dilute my natural hormones did.

At a minimum, an anesthesiologist requires a Liter of IV bolus (comparable to about 4 8oz glasses of water rapidly infused within 30-60 minutes) prior to insertion of an epidural. Once the epidural is in place and as pain is alleviated, the muscles in the walls of blood vessels relax (vasodilation), which often leads to a dramatic drop in blood pressure. Nurses anticipate this shift in blood pressure. In an effort to keep your blood pressure stable and consequently your baby's heart rate stable, we keep the fluids flowing while we take frequent blood pressures. This may mean anywhere from an extra bag of fluid to a few extra bags in a relatively short amount of time.

It is not the intent of your nurse to sabotage your labor by completely diluting the oxytocin out of your bloodstream, but any nurse would rather risk losing your efficient contraction pattern versus risk the wellbeing your baby with the stress of unstable blood pressure.

A mother's hormones obviously play a significant role in labor, but they don't work alone. The hormones work in concert with our muscles and our breath. Deep relaxation that begins with a calm mind will naturally prompt slow, deep breaths and loose muscles. It is important to maintain a loose or relaxed posture throughout labor so that the muscle fibers that comprise the uterus can effectively open the cervix with contractions. The more relaxed the muscles are the more elastic they are.

Oppositely, a strained or tense posture can negatively affect labor as tense muscles result in a tense cervix that resists opening and causes pain. This concept is similar to the pain that arises if tensing the pelvic muscles during a vaginal exam, tampon insertion, or even sex. Conversely, relaxed pelvic muscles promote an elasticity that is capable of accommodating everything from a tampon to your baby's shoulders.

In Childbirth Without Fear, Dr. Grantly Dick-Read writes, "The uterus must be left alone; it can do all this without any effort to help on your part. Consider it a machine apart from yourself, and in due course the dilation of the outlet will be complete. There is no hurry; the door will open, but you must not make the work harder for the uterus by tightening the door. If you are rigid and squeeze up your face, then the muscles of the outlet will squeeze up too. But the uterus is astoundingly strong and persistent; the result of your resistance will be pain. The more completely relaxed you become, so much more elastic will be the mouth of the womb and so much less discomfort with you experience." [7]

I have observed this truth Dr. Grantly Dick-Read describes above and have coached countless laboring mamas to keep their face loose with an open mouth especially during the contraction. This little tip can shave so much discomfort and time off the labor experience.

When we truly let go of our anxieties and tensions and choose softness towards our bodies, we can work with our bodies instead of against them and experience one of the most powerful and beautiful moments of our lives.

Chapter Six
What to Expect During Labor and Helpful Tips

"Birth is not only about making babies. It's about making mothers~ strong, competent, capable mothers who trust themselves and believe in their inner strength."

--Barbara Katz Rothman

It's fascinating how our minds evolve during pregnancy. Often, the birth itself is not something we tend to dwell on during the first trimester. Sure, we may be excited to meet our baby after he or she is born but usually not jazzed for the birthing itself. The thought of pushing a baby out of our body is often just too much to take in, too overwhelming.

As the due date eventually draws near, it's funny how something we avoided thinking about suddenly becomes exciting - something we might pay money to make happen if we could. I remember doing everything in my power to get labor started. Having had sisters, friends, and many pregnant coworkers, I know that I am not the exception.

Having the internet at our fingertips only feeds the insanity. We ask Google the same questions over and over hoping that we will find a sure-fire way to kickstart or "naturally induce" our labors. These suggestions often include castor oil and spicy foods, which are both horrible ideas. A castor oil shot may lead to cramping, but the only thing you'll be delivering is your ensuing diarrhea. Similarly, spicy foods often just lead to heartburn and acid reflux. Other suggestions include sex and nipple stimulation. Fantastic.

Regardless the measures you may try to get things moving, eventually your labor will begin. Labor contractions (different from Braxton Hicks, which are essentially warm-up contractions that practice tightening and releasing your uterine muscles for up to a few hours at a time) typically increase in strength and organize into a pattern. Often contractions start about 20-30 minutes apart and gradually progress to every 15 minutes, then every 10 minutes, etc. While contractions are still somewhat far apart, it is a great time to take a shower or bath, eat something small but nutritious, and make sure you have everything ready that you may need to bring with you if delivering at a birthing facility or hospital. If you are planning a home birth, it is a good time to let your support people know that labor may be starting. This is one very common way that labor begins for a lot of women.

The tricky thing about labor starting with contractions is that sometimes your body may just be practicing or strengthening your uterine muscles. So how do you know what is the real thing and what is just practice when they can seem identical? As mentioned above, real contractions will eventually keep getting closer together and stronger, but sometimes practice contractions mimic this pattern too.

The only way to know for sure is to have your cervix checked. This means going to the Labor and Delivery department to be evaluated for "rule out labor." This can be inconvenient and many women don't want to go to the hospital or birth center if they're just going to be sent home.

My best advice to potentially save you a trip if in fact your body is just in practice mode is to take a bath or shower and drink a large glass of water. Understandably, many women skip this advice because, quite honestly, they want to be in labor so badly that they don't want to risk losing any kind of contraction pattern.

The truth is that real labor will keep progressing no matter what and the more relaxed you can be, the faster this happens. A bath or shower can actually speed things along.

On the flip side, practice contractions will usually subside pretty quickly especially in a warm bath. Getting practice contractions to subside enables you to get some rest and save yourself a trip to the Labor and Delivery department. Another way your body may indicate labor is near is that your amniotic sac (commonly referred to as "water") may break. Only about 15 percent of women's amniotic sac breaks before labor begins. So this is a relatively small tribe but certainly a possibility. Women sometimes assume that the water breaking will be a big obvious gush, but often this isn't the case. It is possible to have a small tear or leak high in the amniotic sac that leads to more of a trickle than a gush. This can be a little trickier to detect.

If you are questioning whether or not your water has broken, it is a good idea to contact your provider and make a plan. Your provider may be concerned about risk of infection if the water is broken for several hours before labor or delivery, as the amniotic sac acts as a protective barrier between outside bacteria and your baby. This is why your labor nurse will check your temperature every couple of hours to detect any early sign of possible infection. If your temperature begins to rise, your provider should talk to you about any concerns he/she may have and any measures that may need to be considered. These measures may include a dose of TYLENOL®, antibiotics, and even augmentation or Pitocin to help speed up the labor before an infection can develop further.

Even if your labor begins with contractions, eventually your water may break on its own or may be broken by your provider. The provider's breaking of your water is another "augmentation" technique that may help speed up labor. Often this technique is suggested somewhere between 3-8 centimeters of dilation. To do this, your nurse or provider will pass what looks like a long skinny plastic crochet hook into your vaginal canal and very carefully tear a small hole in the amniotic sac. This procedure should be quick and painless, but it sometimes takes a couple of tries to tear strong amniotic sacs.

The thinking behind this procedure is that when the water is broken, your baby's head can be applied more directly to the cervix. This results in making each contraction more effective at opening the cervix. Your provider should always have a conversation with you before breaking the water. This is your opportunity to discuss any questions or reservations you may have about it.

Another important amniotic water topic that may come up is its color. If your water breaks before arriving at a facility, one of the first questions you will be asked is, "What color was the fluid?" The fluid can vary between clear and brownish green. The clearer the better. It's important to report any green-colored fluid that you see, as it may signal that your baby needs a little more monitoring for distress. Again, the goal is to have a healthy mom and baby, and your provider and nursing staff want to be aware of any possible risk factors to keep you and your baby as safe and healthy as possible.

Contractions spontaneously starting or your water breaking are the most common and natural starts to labor. However, it is possible that you may be advised to have an induction (the stimulation of uterine contractions with medication prior to natural labor) or even Cesarean section (surgically delivering your baby) for medical reasons. One of the most common reasons to induce early is risk for pre-eclampsia or PIH (pregnancy induced hypertension).

Elevated blood pressure, sudden swelling in your legs, severe headache, epigastric pain (upper abdominal pain), and visual disturbances like seeing spots or blurriness are symptoms to closely monitor. These symptoms generally develop late in pregnancy and typically prompt your provider to order: blood tests, an extended urine collection to check protein levels in the urine over a 24 hour period, and even extra ultrasounds to determine the safety of continuing the pregnancy or if delivery is recommended sooner than later. Most of the time - even if delivery is recommended - an induction will be scheduled, rather than emergency Cesarean section, as often there is time to attempt a vaginal birth rather than an immediate cesarean birth. However, several factors affect this recommendation, and your provider will explain the factors of your specific situation. In extreme cases, a Cesarean section may be recommended (bypassing labor and a vaginal attempt all together) as the safest option for mother and baby. Again, it's important to express any concerns, questions, and reservations to your provider and make a plan together.

Other somewhat common indications for induction may be concern over not having enough amniotic fluid or ample blood supply to your baby through the placenta. Both of these concerns are detected through ultrasound, and your provider will explain in detail the risks and concerns.

Regardless of how your labor begins, eventually you will be on your way to meeting your little one. Active phase of labor is the period of time when your cervix is making significant change in relation to consistent contractions. This is the stage of labor when women typically become more inward focused and often lose awareness of surroundings. This is the stage where modesty often goes out the window, and suddenly it doesn't matter who is in the room or not. This is the stage where you will likely draw upon any prayers, meditations, mantras, visualizations, or other techniques you may have rehearsed.

It is very common to feel an increase of pressure as your baby begins his/her descent and rotates into position to be born. It is best to relax as best you can and actively blow out through your mouth as you exhale to help alleviate the pressure. Pushing too early while you still have cervix left can be counterproductive and cause the remaining cervix to swell. As the pressure increases, your nurse or provider will be at your side to closely monitor cervical changes and check for complete dilation.

If you've decided to have an epidural, the active phase is also the best phase of labor to get it. Early (latent phase) labor can be completely slowed down to a crawl or even stopped if the epidural is given too early. This is usually because of the overload of the bolus of fluids that dilute the little bit of Pitocin your body has released. In this case, likely intravenous (IV) Pitocin will be ordered to help resume labor.

When your cervix is completely dilated, you may begin pushing - especially if you have an urge to push. Experiencing an urge to push is almost always the case without an epidural. Your body knows what to do and is ready to deliver. As each contraction strengthens, so will your natural urge to push as the pressure intensifies. As the contraction begins, you will want to inhale and hold the breath as you focus your push directly into the pressure. Exhale when you need to. With an epidural on board, you may or may not feel pressure or the urge to push. If you do not feel the urge to push, your provider may direct you to continue to rest as your body naturally pushes your baby farther into the birth canal without active pushing from you. An urge to push can be very helpful in directing your efforts. If you can feel the pressure, it is easier to focus energy directly on that pressure as you push.

Without the urge to push, your nurse or provider will help coach you through how to push and give you feedback on your progress. Often this coaching includes directing you to bear down with each contraction. This is a common term in labor and delivery that just means to exert full strength and focused attention when pushing much like pushing to have a bowel movement when constipated. Pregnant women are usually well acquainted with constipation at one time or another during pregnancy, and now all of that experience comes in handy!

When birth is portrayed in movies and in media, the pushing or actual delivery phase of labor seems to be over in minutes. While this is sometimes true, the pushing process more typically may take up to 3-4 hours or longer in some cases.

For first time moms, the average pushing time is a couple of hours. This length of time can actually be helpful in gradually stretching and opening your vaginal canal to reduce tearing. It is important to listen to your body and rest when needed during pushing even if this means breathing through a few contractions versus actively pushing with each one.

Eventually your baby's head will appear, and you will likely be asked if you want to reach down and touch his/her hair for the first time or even watch the progress with a mirror. This is the time when additional staff will be called into the room if needed for a few extra hands when your baby is born. You will also likely be asked if you want your baby placed directly on your chest for immediate skin-to-skin time or dried and wrapped in blankets first.

In certain cases with premature babies or if your amniotic fluid was brown or green with meconium, a nurse practitioner will likely be called to your room to immediately assist your baby with breathing. Often, the nurse practitioner will stand by and wait to see if the baby spontaneously cries before intervening. With more and more education on the benefits of skin-to-skin time, the staff is likely trained to let you hold your baby as soon as possible. This is even true in Cesarean sections. As soon as the baby is stable and breathing on his/her own, the best place for baby to be is skin-to-skin with mom.

Once the baby is delivered and first given to you to hold, this is one of the absolute most precious moments in life. As natural oxytocin hormone is released, you will likely be flooded with a cocktail of emotions of absolute joy, love, relief, and accomplishment. There is nothing like this feeling, and I sincerely hope that you relish every moment of it. Congratulations!

Chapter Seven
Prayers, Meditations, and Mantras

"Silence isn't empty, it's full of answers."

--Unknown

This chapter is intended to be a practice guide for the active phase of labor. For women desiring a natural birth without an epidural, I strongly encourage contemplating and practicing strategies that would be helpful to you in labor to halt fear and anxiety in their tracks. I strongly believe that having a strong mind and choosing your thoughts will serve you well through labor as well as through life in general.

With that said, not every technique is for everyone, and that's ok. The key is to be mindful about what resonates with you personally. Use the prayers, meditations, mantras, and visualizations below, or feel free to create your own. These positive words or visualizations - when practiced frequently - will help create pathways in your brain. Then when labor comes, your mind can easily choose these paths that are calm and safe, rather than be overtaken by thoughts of anxiety, control, and fear. I wish you a joyous birth experience and hope that you find renewed strength in yourself through this journey.

PRAYERS AND SCRIPTURES

Thank you for the blessing of being pregnant and the opportunity to share in the joy of the life you are creating in me. I give you my anxieties, worries, and even expectations of the birth of this precious child. I ask that you be with me and strengthen me. I ask that you keep my baby and me safe and healthy. I trust you. Amen.
******

Thank you for the miracle you are creating in me. Thank you for life itself. I ask for your peace and guidance as I embark on this new journey.

Philippians 4:13 "I can do all things through Christ who strengthens me."

Psalm 91:1-2 "He who dwells in the shelter of the Most High will abide in the shadow of the Almighty. I will say to the Lord, "My refuge and my fortress, my God, in whom I trust."

Psalm 121:1-3 "I lift up my eyes to the mountains— where does my help come from? My help comes from the Lord, the Maker of heaven and earth. He will not let your foot slip— he who watches over you will not slumber."

Isaiah 41:10 "Do not fear, for I am with you; do not be dismayed, for I am your God. I will strengthen you and help you; I will uphold you with my righteous right hand."

Isaiah 43:1-2 "Do not fear, for I have redeemed you; I have called you by name; you are mine. When you pass through the waters, I will be with you; and through the rivers, they shall not overwhelm you; when you walk through fire you shall not be burned, and the flame shall not consume you."

Philippians 4:8 "Whatever is true, whatever is noble, whatever is right, whatever is pure, whatever is lovely, whatever is admirable—if anything is excellent or praiseworthy—think about such things."

MANTRAS

(These mantras are meant to be repeated on a daily basis. They can be recited and practiced while resting, meditating, or even when waiting in line at the grocery store. They are simple but positive thoughts to help create a strong and healthy mind.)

I am strong.

I trust my body.

I am relaxed and safe.

My baby will be born in calm and love.

I breathe in. I breathe out.

I let go of control.

I am enough.

Today is a day of happiness and peace.

I am completely at peace.

I am grounded and centered.

I let go of fear.

My body is completely capable of birth.

I release and relax.

The pressure is intense, but my body was made for this.

My baby and I are working together.

I am confident.

One breath at a time.

My body is incredible.

My body knows exactly how and when to birth my baby.

May I be well. May I be happy. May I be free from suffering.

May my baby be well. May my baby be happy. May my baby be free from suffering.

MEDITATIONS AND VISUALIZATIONS

Find a safe, calm, and quiet space. I recommend sitting upright with your back supported and your eyes closed as you practice these techniques. It is perfectly normal for the mind to wander - especially if you are new to any sort of meditation practice. With repetition, your mind will get stronger and have a longer and longer capacity to focus on your breath or visualization that you choose. Below are three meditations that progress from basic and breath-focused to symbolic and reflective visualizations.

Place your hands on your belly as you sit with a slight grin or smile. Spend a minute or two focusing on your breath alone. Feel your belly expand as you inhale and fall as you exhale. Slowly and gradually slow your breath as you focus on the sensation of breathing. When settled in, now visualize a warm golden light at the base of your spine warming your baby. Continue focusing on this light and basking in its warm radiant glow. If your mind begins to wander, gently return to focus on the gradual rise and fall of your belly as you breathe.

I am like a tree. I am grounded with deep roots that sustain me. I have everything that I need. My trunk is strong as I stretch up to the sky. Even when the winds are strong, I will not be moved. My branches reach far into the sky to provide shade and comfort for those who look to me for refuge. I even provide fruit for those under my care. I have everything I need and more. Out of abundance I give to those around me. My branches are strong yet flexible just like me. I withstand the storms by swaying with the winds rather than fighting against them.

****

I visualize myself barefoot walking up a riverbank. It is summer and the water is perfectly warm. The stones under my feet are smooth. I hear the sound of gently flowing water and the chirping of birds in the distance. The sunshine is on my back and fills me with warmth and light. As I walk, I hold an apron with a few stones I have been carrying along the way. Some of them I have been carrying for years, some of them large, some of them small. As I walk through the water, I realize I do not need these stones any longer. I have carried them far enough. I slowly and purposefully place each stone back into the stream. These stones represent doubt, fear, a grudge held, a person I have judged or not forgiven, and insecurities. With each stone I drop, I feel peace settling within me. Joy is stirred up from my belly and I embrace everything around me just as it is. I embrace myself just as I am and let go of my desire for approval and pleasing. I know that I am wonderfully made and that I am good. I am free. I am well.

I hope that this book has provided a pathway to a more confident, centered, and ultimately joyous pregnancy and birth. Thank you for sharing your time and energy with me as you prepare for this exciting journey. I sincerely hope you have found helpful tips and feel a little more prepared for what to expect. May you have an overwhelming sense that you were made for this incredible privilege of motherhood.

Bibliography

"[1] Charles Dickens, A Tale of Two Cities , 1859 (reprint,Mineola, N.Y.: Dover Thrift Editions, 1999),

[2] American College of Obstetricians and Gynecologists, https://www.acog.org/-/media/womens-health/nutrition-in-pregnancy.pdf , 320.

[3] Luther, M. (1998). By faith alone: 365 devotional readings updated in today's language . Iowa City, IA: World Bible Publishers

[4] Marie Mongan, (2005). Hypnobirthing The Mongan Method , (3rd Edition). Health Communications, Inc.

[5] Rea Nolan Martin (2013). How to Feed the Body, Mind, and Spirit. https://www.huffpost.com/entry/body-mind-spirit_b_4240886

[6] Lindsey Welch (2017). Birth Hormones and Feeling Safe During Labor , lindseywelchchildbirtheducator.wordpress.com,

[7] Dr. Grantly Dick-Read (2013). Childbirth Without Fear , Pinter & Martin Ltd."